GUT-BRAIN THERAPY

Therapies For Mood Regulation And Mental Health

Explore The Connection Between Gut Health And Mental Well-Being, With Therapeutic Strategies For A Balanced Mind

DR. BRIDGET PROMISE

Table of Contents

CHAPTER ONE

Introduction

The complex interplay between the gastrointestinal tract and the brain is an intriguing and dynamic field of scientific investigation.

Beyond the conventional comprehension of the digestive system's function in metabolizing food, recent studies have illuminated the profound influence of the gastrointestinal tract on psychological well-being.

Frequently denoted the "gut-brain axis," this link between the central nervous system and the gastrointestinal tract entails an intricate interplay of signals. This investigation examines the fundamental ramifications of the gut-brain relationship, with a specific emphasis on the impact of dietary patterns on mental health, the significance of probiotics and prebiotics in promoting emotional well-being, and the function of gut microbiota.

Comprehending The Fibre-Brain Interplay:

The gut-brain connection is a reciprocal web of communication that spans from the central nervous system (CNS) to the enteric nervous system (ENS), also known as the "second brain." Consisting of an intricate network of neurons that line the gastrointestinal tract, the ENS is vital for controlling absorption, digestion, and overall gut functionality.

Multiple pathways facilitate communication between the intestine and the brain, encompassing the vagus nerve, hormones, and mediators of the immune system.

The Function Of Gut Microbiota In The Regulation Of Mood

The gut-brain connection is fundamentally influenced by the gut microbiota, an intricate community comprising trillions of microorganisms that reside within the digestive tract.

The microbiota comprises various microorganisms, including bacteria, viruses, fungi, and others, which collectively form the microbial ecosystem of the intestine. The composition and diversity of this microbiota are crucial factors in determining the regulation of temperament and emotional well-being, among other aspects of human health.

The gut microbiota is capable of producing mood-regulating neurotransmitters, including serotonin and dopamine, according to scientific research.

Serotonin, a neurotransmitter frequently called the "feel-good" neurotransmitter, plays a crucial role in the control of appetite, sleep, and mood. An estimated ninety percent of serotonin is synthesized in the gastrointestinal tract. There is evidence linking disturbances in the equilibrium of gut microbiota to mood disorders, such as anxiety and depression.

Dietary Influence On Mental Health

The effects of dietary decisions on both gastrointestinal health and mental well-being are profound. A varied and unprocessed food selection facilitates the absorption of vital nutrients that promote the development and upkeep of a balanced intestinal microbiota.

A diet high in processed foods, fructose, and saturated lipids, on the other hand, can disrupt the microbial balance in the intestines.

Research has linked the Mediterranean diet, which is distinguished by its substantial intake of fruits, vegetables, whole cereals, and healthy lipids, to a reduced likelihood of developing melancholy and cognitive decline.

A contrast is the association between low-fiber, refined-sugar diets and an elevated risk of developing mental health disorders.

CHAPTER TWO

The Impact Of Probiotics On Emotional Well-Being:

Probiotics are viable microorganisms, predominantly advantageous bacteria, which bestow advantageous effects on health when ingested in sufficient quantities.

Besides supplements, these microorganisms are present in fermented foods such as kefir, kimchi, yogurt, and sauerkraut. Probiotics are of paramount importance in regulating the intestinal microbiota composition and fostering a harmonious equilibrium of microorganisms.

A multitude of scholarly investigations have examined the capacity of probiotics to impact emotional well-being. Several probiotic strains, including Bifidobacterium and Lactobacillus, have been linked to a decrease in depressive and anxious symptoms.

The mechanisms by which this effect is exerted involve neurotransmitter synthesis, inflammation regulation, and the preservation of a healthy intestinal barrier.

Sustaining The Gut With Prebiotics To Promote Mental Health

Although probiotics are the subject of substantial discussion, prebiotics hold an equivalent level of significance in promoting digestive health. Prebiotics are a class of nondigestible fibers that provide nourishment for advantageous intestinal microbiota. Prebiotics are frequently found in fruits, vegetables, whole cereals, and legumes.

Prebiotics contribute to the synthesis of short-chain fatty acids (SCFAs), which are essential for gut health maintenance and have a significant impact on the gut-brain axis, through the nourishment of the gut microbiota. It is well-established that SCFAs maintain the integrity of the intestinal barrier and possess anti-inflammatory properties.

Preventing the passage of hazardous substances from the gastrointestinal tract into the circulation, which may have adverse effects on the central nervous system, requires a robust intestinal barrier.

The critical relationship between the stomach and the brain underscores the significance of promoting digestive health to enhance overall wellness. The gut-brain axis is characterized by an intricate web of communication, in which the gut microbiota exerts a pivotal influence on affective well-being and mood.

The importance of conscientiously selecting foods to promote brain and gastrointestinal health is driven home by the correlation between diet and mental health.

Moreover, through their ability to nourish the gut microbiota, prebiotics facilitate the synthesis of advantageous compounds that exert a positive impact on the gut-brain axis.

With the ongoing development of knowledge regarding the relationship between the gut and the brain, it becomes more pertinent to incorporate gut health-promoting practices, such as a well-balanced diet abundant in probiotics and prebiotics, to enhance emotional resilience and mental well-being.

By acknowledging and embracing the reciprocal association between the gastrointestinal tract and the brain, we establish a foundation for comprehensive wellness that investigates the physical and emotional dimensions of health.

Recent years have witnessed an increased recognition of the complex relationship between gastrointestinal health and mental health.

The notion of gut-brain harmony underscores the significant influence that a range of lifestyle components—including but not limited to diet, mindfulness, exercise, sleep hygiene, and herbal remedies—can exert on the digestive system and mental health.

A Natural Approach To Gut-Brain Harmony Via Fermented Foods

Fermented foods have been dietary components of human beings for numerous centuries, renowned for their distinctive qualities as well as the potential health advantages they offer.

This gastronomic custom incorporates the organic fermentation procedure, during which food constituents are decomposed by microorganisms such as yeast, bacteria, and molds into novel compounds. A critical consequence of this process is the proliferation of probiotics, which are advantageous bacteria recognized for their ability to foster a healthy intestinal microbiome.

Fermented Nutrients Are Highly Significant In Gut-Brain Harmony. The community of microorganisms known as the gut microbiome, which is found in the digestive tract, exerts a substantial influence on both cognitive processes and psychological well-being.

Probiotics facilitate the maintenance of the microbiome's equilibrium by cultivating a milieu that is favorable for the synthesis of neurotransmitters, including serotonin, which is commonly known as the "happy hormone."

Consuming fermented foods, including kombucha, sauerkraut, kefir, yogurt, and kimchi, can be a delectable and natural way to promote digestive health. Fermented foods positively impact mental health by fostering a harmonious intestinal microbiome, thereby contributing to a positive feedback cycle.

CHAPTER THREE

Cultivating Awareness For Mental Wellness Through Mindful Eating

In addition to the physical act of ingesting food, the concept of mindful eating entails devoting one's complete concentration to the entirety of the dining experience.

By cultivating an awareness of the present moment, mindful dining promotes an appreciation for the visual, tactile, and gustatory aspects of every morsel.

By adopting this method, one not only amplifies the gustatory pleasure derived from dining but also forges a deep correlation between the physical and mental realms.

Regarding the harmony between the stomach and the brain, mindful dining enhances one's awareness and understanding of food.

By developing an awareness of their appetite and satiety signals, people can avoid excess and facilitate efficient digestion. Additionally, practicing mindful dining cultivates an attitude of appreciation for the sustenance one has ingested, thereby fostering a constructive frame of mind that may permeate other facets of existence.

Herbal Remedies To Promote Gut-Brain Harmony

Herbal remedies with a traditional origin have been utilized to treat a wide range of health issues, including those affecting the gut and brain, for centuries. Herbs are known to contain naturally occurring compounds that have the potential to improve both digestive and mental health.

Several botanicals, including chamomile, peppermint, and ginger, have been linked to advantageous effects on digestion.

For instance, peppermint is recognized for its capacity to alleviate gastrointestinal distress, whereas ginger possesses anti-nausea attributes. Because of its tranquil properties, chamomile may aid in tension reduction and sleep improvement.

Ashwagandha and holy basil are examples of adaptogenic botanicals renowned for their capacity to assist the body in adjusting to stress. Effective stress management is of paramount importance in promoting balance between the gut and brain, given that persistent stress can have detrimental effects on the gut microbiome and potentially contribute to mental health disorders.

By integrating herbal remedies, such as beverages, tinctures, or supplements, into one's wellness regimen, a natural and holistic strategy can be established to bolster the equilibrium between the gastrointestinal tract and the brain.

The Positive Impact Of Physical Activity On Mental Health

It has long been acknowledged that physical activity is beneficial for both physical and mental health. Consistent physical activity not only enhances cardiovascular fitness and aids in weight management but also significantly contributes to the promotion of mental well-being.

Within the realm of gut-brain harmony, research has demonstrated that physical activity can impact the diversity and composition of the gut microbiome. The proliferation of beneficial microbes can be increased through physical activity, thereby promoting a more salubrious intestinal environment.

Often referred to as the gut-brain axis, exercise has been found to positively impact the communication between the intestines and brain, which may have implications for the potential reduction of mental health disorders.

Furthermore, physical activity is an effective method of reducing tension. Participating in physical exercise stimulates the secretion of endorphins, which are endogenous tension alleviations. Physical activity indirectly promotes a symbiotic relationship between the brain and stomach by mitigating stress.

The Importance Of Sleep Hygiene In Mood Regulation

Sufficient sleep is critical for optimal health, and its significance is further compounded by the complex interplay between the gastrointestinal tract and the brain. Sleep hygiene, which consists of routines and practices that facilitate deeper, higher-quality sleep, is an indispensable component in mood regulation and mental health support.

Insomnia and irregular sleep patterns are examples of sleep disturbances that can impair the equilibrium of the gastrointestinal microbiome. Existing research indicates that sleep deprivation may result in a disruption of gut microbiota, which could potentially be a contributing factor to the development of gastrointestinal disorders such as irritable bowel syndrome (IBS).

In contrast, a state of optimal gut microbiome health can have a beneficial impact on sleep patterns and enhance the overall quality of sleep.

Promoting proper sleep hygiene entails establishing a sleeping environment that is conducive to rest, adhering to regular sleep regimens, and incorporating relaxation techniques before nighttime. Promoting optimal sleep quality can facilitate the complex interaction between the gastrointestinal tract and the brain, thereby nurturing mental health as a whole.

In summary, the notion of gut-brain harmony emphasizes the importance of lifestyle elements in impacting psychological and gastrointestinal well-being. In addition to prioritizing sleep hygiene and incorporating fermented foods and mindful dining, herbal remedies, and regular exercise are all vital components of a holistic approach to health. By cultivating a harmonious intestinal microbiome and embracing mindful practices, individuals can initiate a process that contributes to enhanced mental well-being and holistic health.

CHAPTER FOUR

Techniques Of Stress Management For A Healthier Gut-Brain Axis

In our contemporary society, characterized by rapidity and change, tension has virtually become an inevitable component of existence. The pervasive influence of stress on our holistic well-being extends beyond our mental health to encompass the intricate equilibrium of the gut-brain axis.

The correlation between the gastrointestinal tract and the brain is vital for the preservation of both physical and mental well-being. The establishment of efficient stress management strategies is critical in promoting the well-being of the gut-brain axis.

The implementation of techniques that assist the body and mind in coping with and mitigating stressors constitutes stress management.

It has been demonstrated that practices such as mindfulness meditation, deep breathing exercises, and consistent physical activity have a beneficial effect on the gut-brain axis. Effective stress management enables the intestine to preserve its microbial equilibrium, thereby fostering a symbiotic association with the brain.

Integrity Of The Gut And Brain In Neurological Disorders

In contemporary scientific discourse, the importance of the gut-brain axis in a multitude of neurological disorders has become progressively more apparent.

Schizophrenia, Parkinson's disease, and multiple sclerosis are among the conditions that have been associated with changes in the intestinal microbiota. The gut-brain axis, a complex network of communication connecting the gut and brain, is involved in the regulation of immune responses and inflammation, both of which are implicated in the pathogenesis and advancement of these conditions.

The comprehension of the gut-brain axis's function in neurological disorders presents novel opportunities for prospective therapeutic interventions. Probiotics and prebiotics, which seek to regulate the intestinal microbiota, are being investigated as supplementary treatments to conventional methods for the management of these conditions. Through investigating the relationship between the stomach and the brain, scientists aspire to discover innovative approaches that can enhance the quality of life for those afflicted with neurological disorders.

Supportive Nutritional Supplements For Mental Health

As a result of the sensitivity of the gut-brain axis to nutritional factors, specific supplements may contribute to mental health support. Fish oil contains omega-3 fatty acids, which have been linked to mood regulation and cognitive function. By contributing to the structural integrity of brain cell membranes, these essential fatty acids affect the function of neurotransmitters.

Furthermore, probiotics, which are advantageous microorganisms, have exhibited potential in promoting psychological well-being. Probiotics contribute to the regulation of intestinal microbiota, exerting an impact on the synthesis of neurotransmitters such as serotonin, which is commonly known as the "feel-good" neurotransmitter. Furthermore, the integration of a wide array of nutrients, including vitamins and minerals, serves to bolster the gut-brain axis and promote holistic mental health.

Harmony Of The Gut And Brain In Children And Adolescents

The gut-brain axis assumes a critical role, especially in the developmental stages of childhood and adolescence. Disruptions to the gastrointestinal microbiota during the period of brain development may result in enduring consequences for both physical and mental well-being. Therefore, the overall health of infants and adolescents must promote gut-brain harmony.

Advocating for the consumption of a well-rounded and nourishing diet is fundamental in fostering optimal gut-brain function among adolescents.

The consumption of foods abundant in fiber, prebiotics, and probiotics promotes the proliferation of advantageous intestinal microbiota. Furthermore, by incorporating stress management techniques into their curriculum and encouraging them to participate in consistent physical activity, educators can furnish young individuals with invaluable resources to sustain a robust gut-brain connection while they confront the complexities of maturation.

CHAPTER FIVE

Investigating The Connection Between Gut Health And Anxiety

A prevalent mental health issue, anxiety has been linked near the gut-brain axis. Due to the bidirectional communication between the intestines and the brain, anxiety disorders may be exacerbated or developed in part as a result of digestive health disturbances.

On the contrary, chronic anxiety has the potential to perturb the microbial composition and function of the intestine.

Exploring the correlation between gastrointestinal health and anxiety presents novel opportunities for the development of holistic strategies aimed at managing anxiety. Lifestyle interventions that emphasize digestive health, including modifications to one's diet and techniques for reducing stress, have the potential to supplement conventional therapeutic approaches for anxiety disorders.

Furthermore, investigations into psychobiotics, which are probiotics with a specific impact on mental health, are providing insights into the potential efficacy of these advantageous microbes in mitigating anxiety symptoms.

In summary, the gut-brain axis is a complex and dynamic system that is essential for the maintenance of general well-being.

The implementation of stress management strategies, including engaging in physical activity and practicing mindfulness, can positively influence the gut-brain axis by alleviating the physiological effects of stress. The correlation between the intestine and the brain is of specific significance in the context of neurological disorders, as therapeutic approaches that focus on the gut microbiota may have the potential to enhance patient prognoses.

Supplementary nutrients, particularly probiotics and omega-3 fatty acids, have the potential to promote mental well-being through their impact on neurotransmitter activity and maintenance of a harmonious intestinal microbiota.

It is of the utmost importance to promote gut-brain harmony in infants and adolescents by emphasizing stress management, physical activity, and nutrition. In conclusion, the correlation between anxiety and digestive health underscores the need for a comprehensive approach to mental well-being that incorporates lifestyle modifications that emphasize maintaining a healthy stomach-brain axis.

By recognizing and fostering this complex correlation, individuals can adopt proactive measures to attain their utmost physical and mental health.

Therapeutic Strategies Employing The Gut Microbiome In The Context Of Depression

The correlation between the intestinal microbiome and mental health has become an area of increasing scholarly attention and investigation in recent times.

Conventional methods of managing depression frequently encompass psychological interventions and pharmacotherapy. However, the burgeoning discipline of gut-brain connection investigates the potential impact of the gut microbiome on psychological health. The aforementioned paradigm shift has given rise to novel therapeutic methodologies that seek to exploit the relationship between the stomach and brain to enhance cognition and mental well-being.

Leveraging The Binomial-Brain Interplay To Boost Cognitive Performance

The gut-brain connection pertains to the reciprocal exchange of information between the brain and the intestine, which is facilitated by the gut microbiome—a heterogeneous assemblage of microorganisms that inhabit the digestive tract. This mutualistic association is of paramount importance in preserving holistic health, encompassing psychological wellness. Important mood and cognition regulators include neurotransmitters such as serotonin and dopamine, which are produced by the gastrointestinal microbiome.

Therapeutic strategies that target the relationship between the intestines and the brain optimize the balance of beneficial microbes in the gut to improve mental health. Probiotics, a class of living microorganisms that may confer health advantages, have garnered considerable interest due to their ability to regulate the intestinal microbiome. Research indicates that specific strains of probiotics might alleviate symptoms of depression and exert a positive influence on mood.

Furthermore, research is being conducted to determine whether prebiotics—substances that stimulate the development of beneficial bacteria—can improve mental health.

Prebiotics foster the growth and development of beneficial

microorganisms by providing the intestinal microbiome with the proper nutrients. Consequently, this could potentially lead to enhanced temperament and cognitive performance.

Case Studies: Actual Metamorphoses Induced By Gut-Brain Therapies

Case studies from real life provide convincing evidence that gut-brain therapies can effectively treat depression. Those afflicted with protracted depressive symptoms frequently discover that conventional treatments offer only modest alleviation.

Interventions that focus on the gastrointestinal microbiome present renewed optimism and potential for progress in such circumstances.

Consider Sarah, a 35-year-old woman who had endured a protracted battle with melancholy. The efficacy of conventional treatments had been limited, prompting her to explore alternative methodologies. After researching gut-brain therapies, Sarah integrated prebiotics and probiotics into her daily regimen.

She gradually documented a discernible enhancement in her emotional state, vitality, and general state of being. The transition encompassed alterations at the microbial level as well as psychological ones, underscoring the complex interaction between the gastrointestinal tract and the brain.

In a similar vein, James, a 45-year-old male who was experiencing treatment-resistant depression, had his entire intestinal microbiome analyzed. The findings informed a customized strategy that integrated particular probiotics and dietary modifications to foster a more salubrious intestinal milieu. Over the subsequent months, James underwent a substantial amelioration of his depressive symptoms, thereby demonstrating the potential of gut-brain interventions that are specifically designed to address individual requirements.

CHAPTER SIX

The Prospects For Gut-Brain Therapies And Research

The ongoing progress in gut-brain research bodes well for the development of personalized and more targeted therapies in the future.

The investigation of psychobiotics, which are probiotics that have positive effects on mental health, is an uncharted domain in which researchers strive to identify strains that influence mood and cognition in particular. By taking into account the specific composition of an individual's gastrointestinal microbiome, precision medicine methodologies have the potential to inform customized interventions that yield improved outcomes.

Technological advancements, including artificial intelligence and microbiome sequencing, are anticipated to have a significant impact on elucidating the intricate dynamics of the gut-brain connection.

Enhanced comprehension in this area may pave the way for the creation of innovative therapeutic approaches, such as fecal microbiota transplantation and microbial-based interventions, which aim to modify the gut microbiome and mitigate symptoms associated with depression.

Conclusion

In conclusion, holistic well-being can be attained by achieving gut-brain balance.

The investigation into the relationship between the stomach and the brain has revealed novel approaches to treating depression and fostering holistic health. Although conventional treatments continue to hold merit, the incorporation of gut-centric methodologies presents a supplementary and potentially paradigm-shifting aspect to the field of mental health.

Achieving gut-brain balance necessitates the implementation of a comprehensive strategy that includes lifestyle adjustments, probiotic and prebiotic supplementation, and dietary modifications.

By adopting these interventions, individuals may experience a reduction in depressive symptoms and develop greater cognitive and emotional resilience.

Further exploration of the complex interaction between the gastrointestinal tract and the brain is transforming the therapeutic terrain for depression. To fully harness the potential of gut-brain therapies, it is imperative that researchers, healthcare professionals, and individuals seeking mental health support work in concert.

By cultivating an all-encompassing comprehension of wellness that incorporates physiological and psychological aspects, we can lay the groundwork for a future in which individuals are enabled to reclaim their mental health and lead satisfying lives through the use of individualized, efficacious, and groundbreaking treatments.

www.ingramcontent.com/pod-product-compliance
Lightning Source LLC
Chambersburg PA
CBHW070723260726
48660CB00007B/2693